# THE DISCOVER CATS
## EXPLORE FAMOUS INVENTIONS

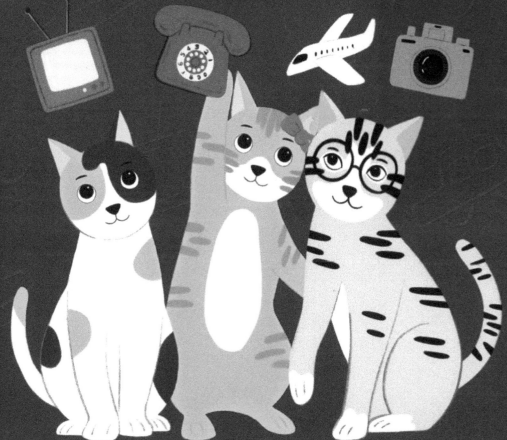

Written by Jimmy Nightingale -- Illustrated by Grace Ji

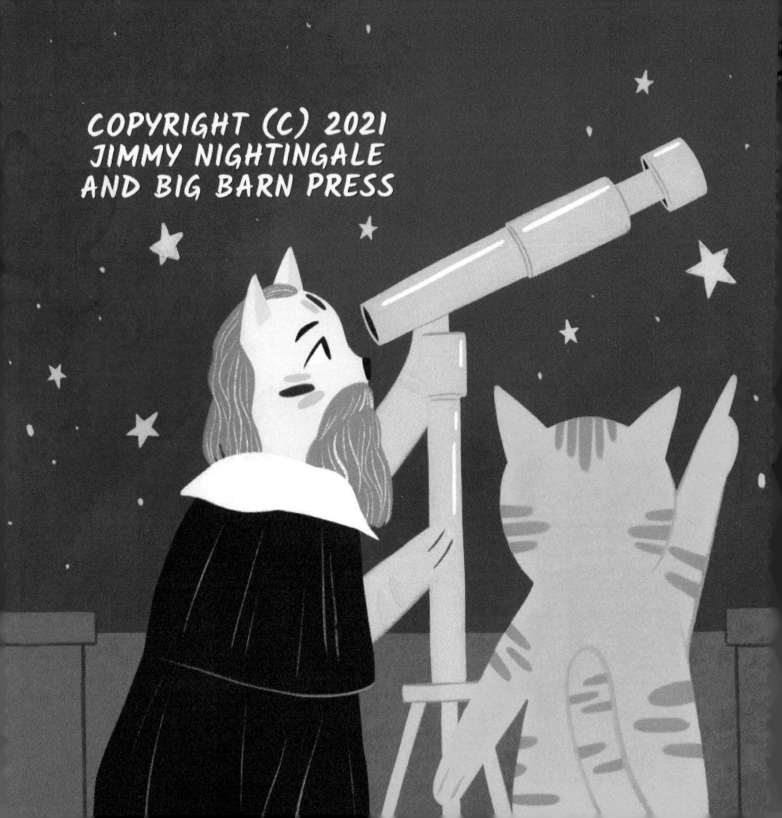

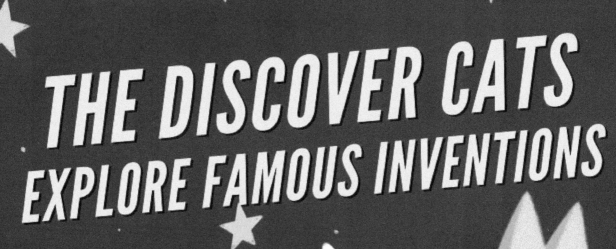

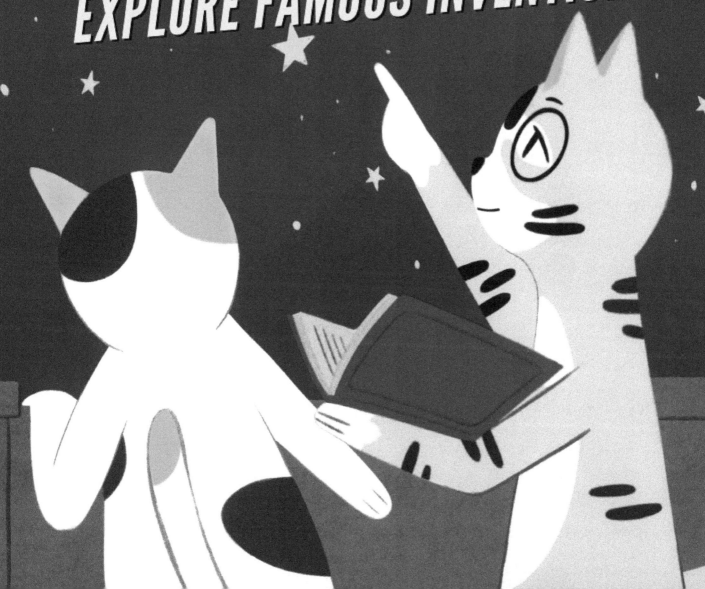

Ginny and Max were playing with their toy trains and cars one day. Rawr! Max was winning! Ginny asked, "Max, where do cars come from?" Max didn't know!

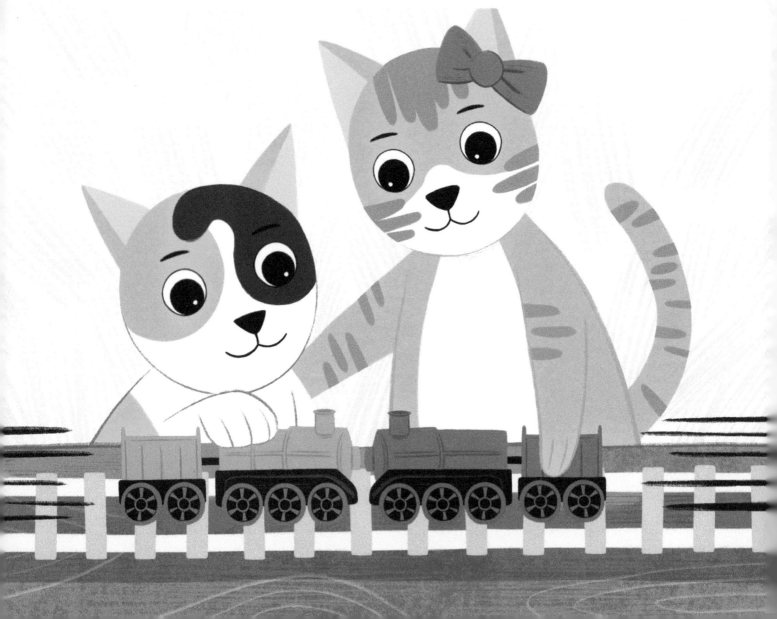

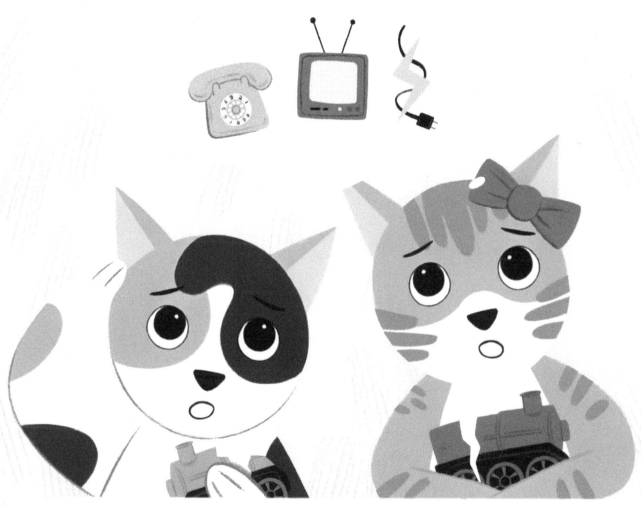

They started wondering where all the other things they used came from. The lights in their house, their books, the internet, their list was fast expanding!

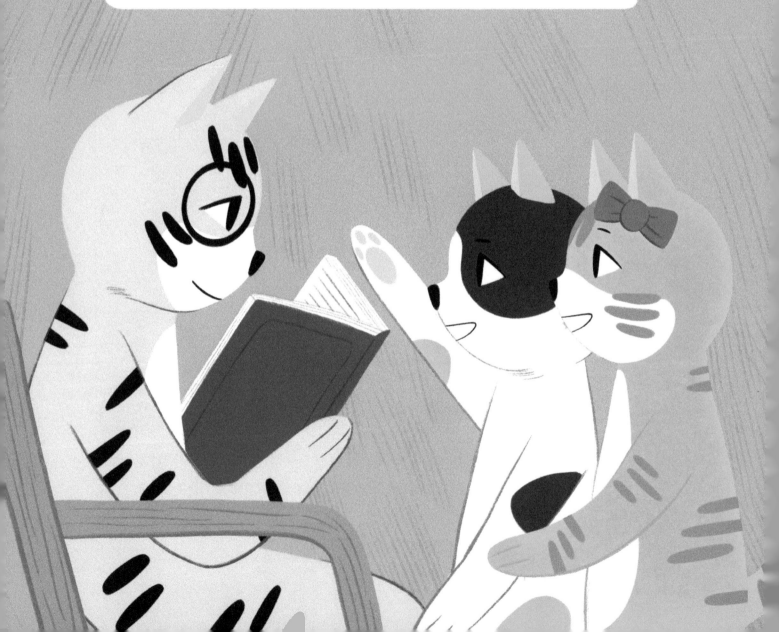

It was time to ask the smartest cat they knew: their older brother, Cornelius.

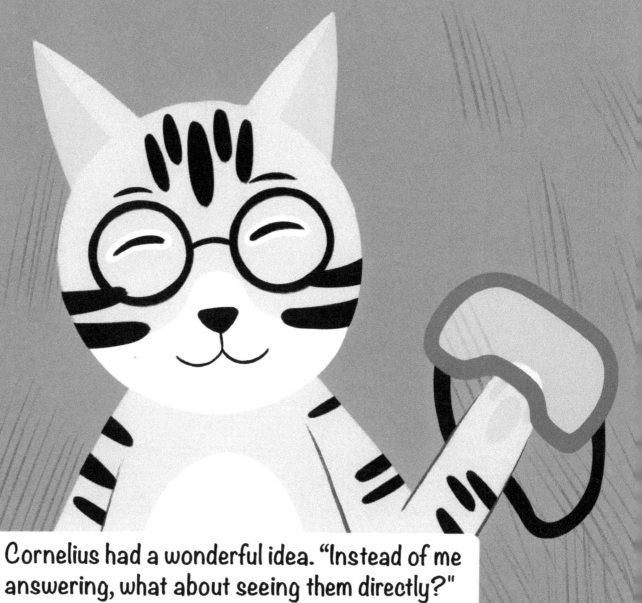

Cornelius had a wonderful idea. "Instead of me answering, what about seeing them directly?"

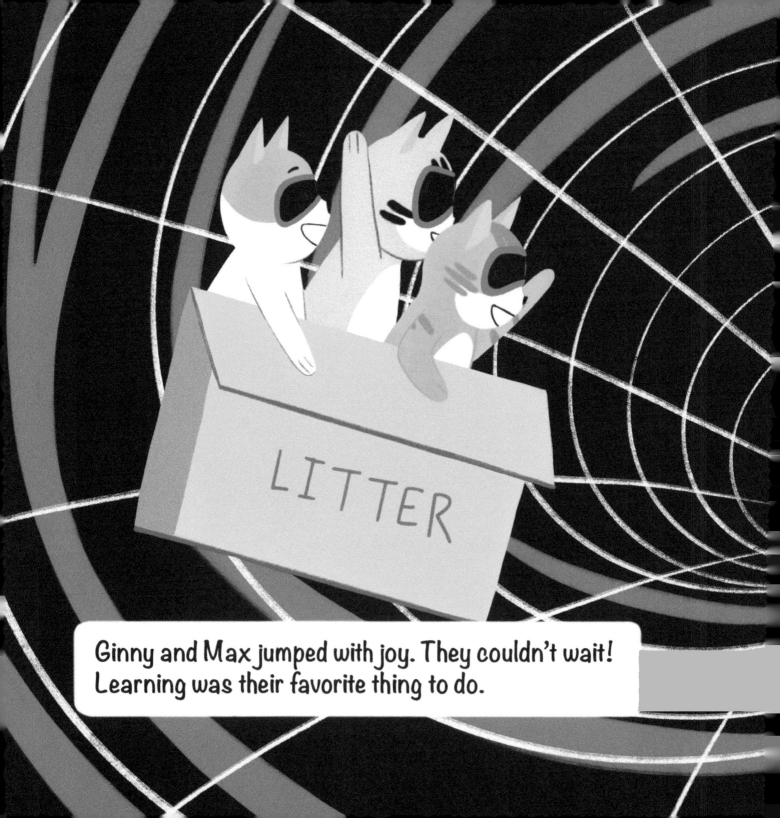

Ginny and Max jumped with joy. They couldn't wait! Learning was their favorite thing to do.

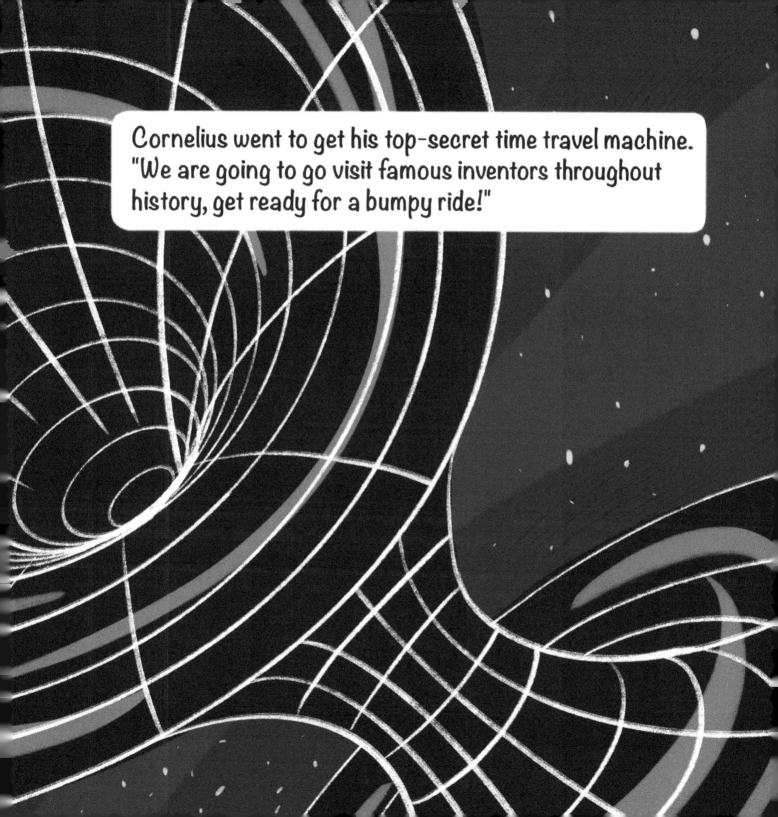

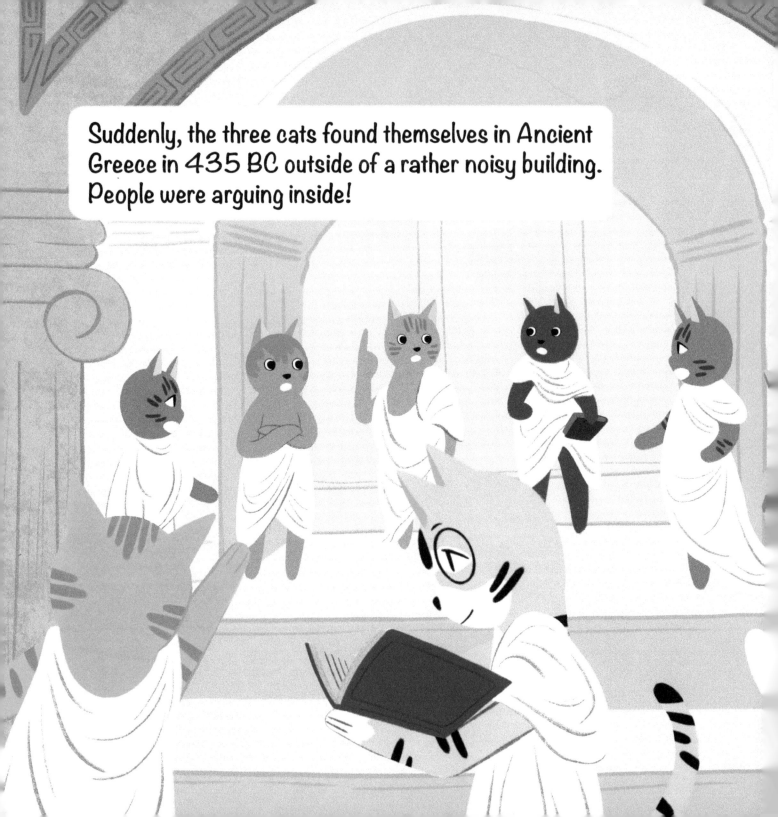

Suddenly, the three cats found themselves in Ancient Greece in 435 BC outside of a rather noisy building. People were arguing inside!

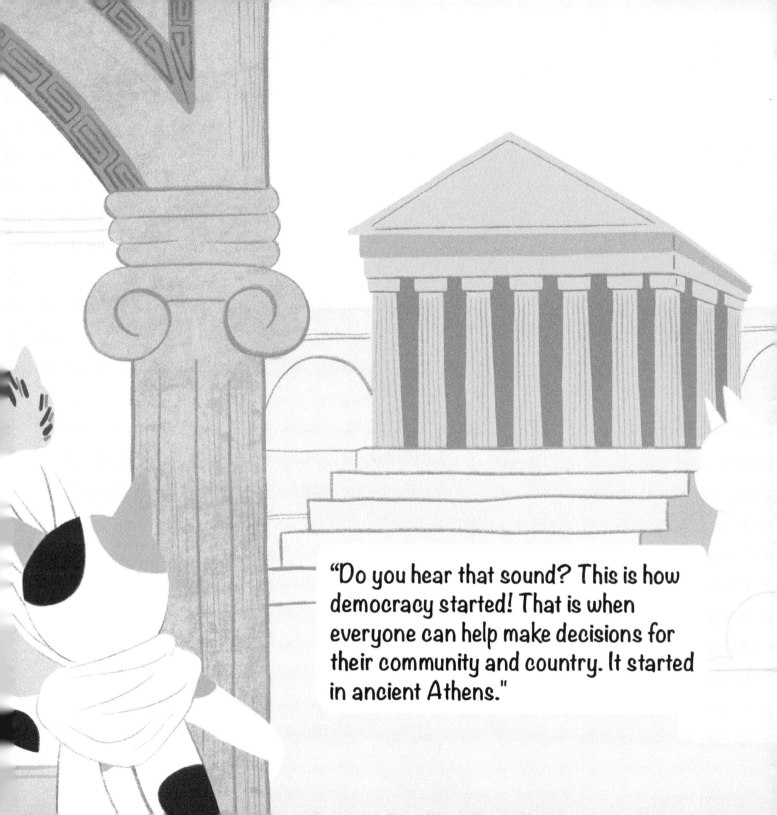

"Do you hear that sound? This is how democracy started! That is when everyone can help make decisions for their community and country. It started in ancient Athens."

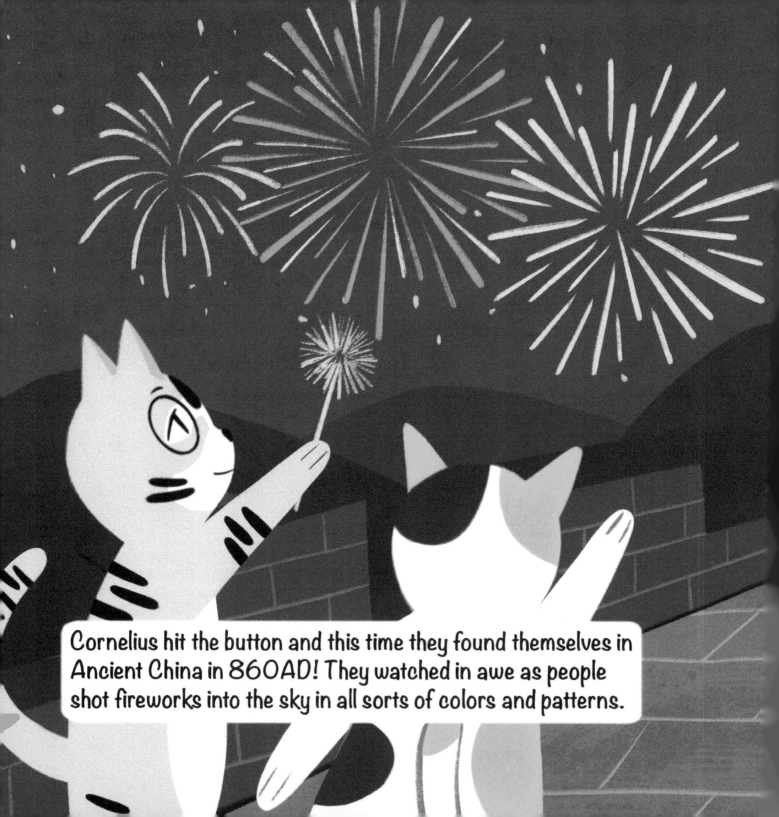

Cornelius hit the button and this time they found themselves in Ancient China in 860AD! They watched in awe as people shot fireworks into the sky in all sorts of colors and patterns.

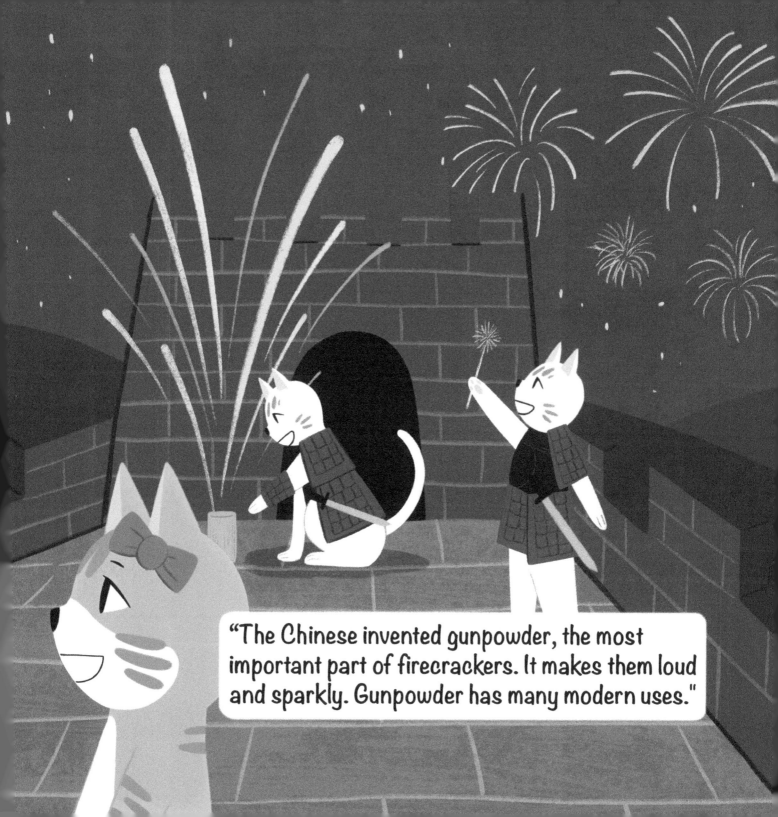

"The Chinese invented gunpowder, the most important part of firecrackers. It makes them loud and sparkly. Gunpowder has many modern uses."

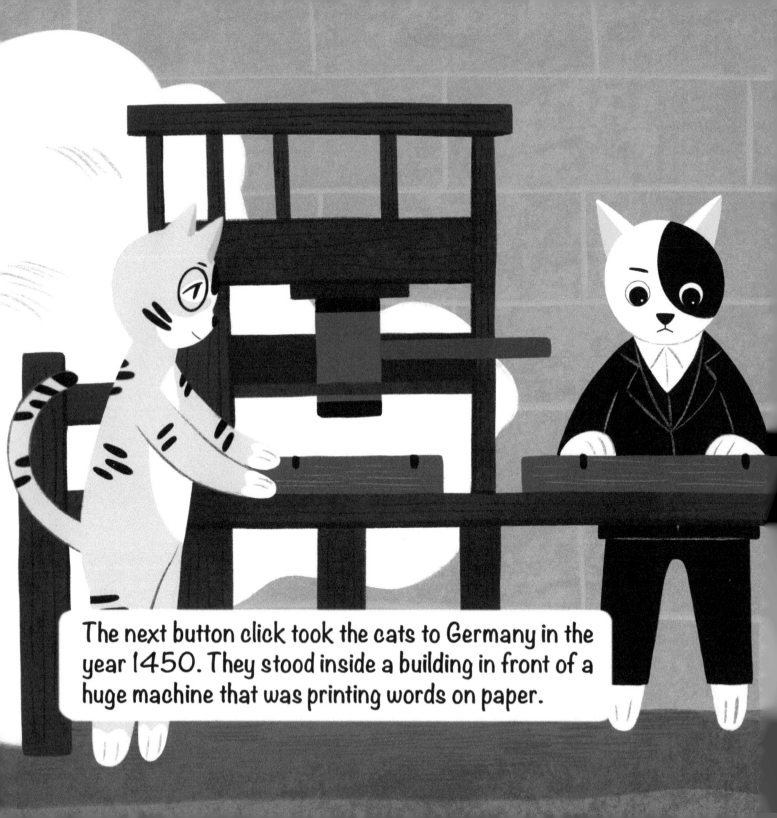

The next button click took the cats to Germany in the year 1450. They stood inside a building in front of a huge machine that was printing words on paper.

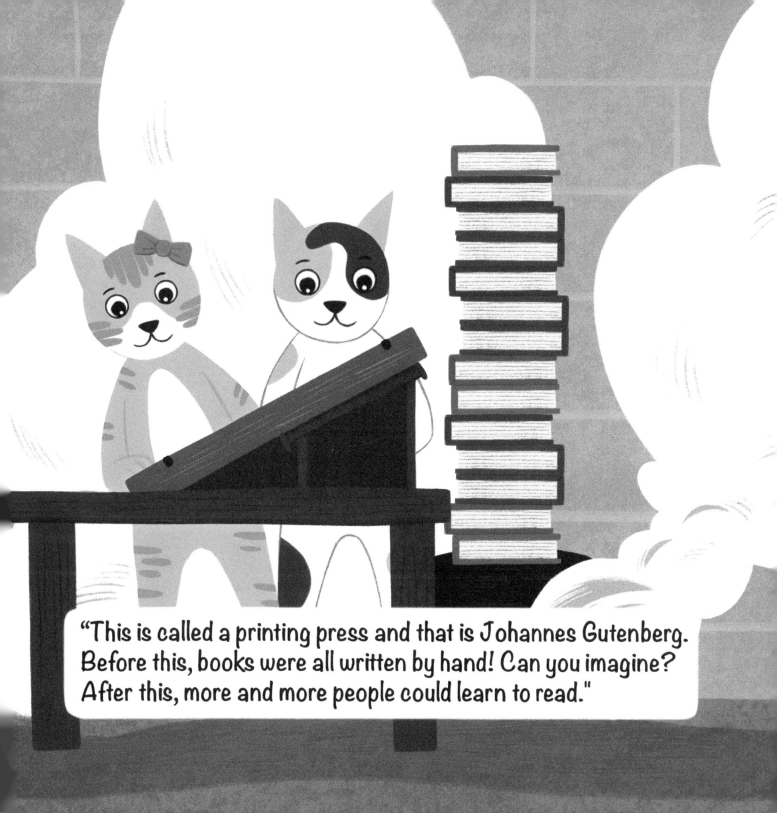

"This is called a printing press and that is Johannes Gutenberg. Before this, books were all written by hand! Can you imagine? After this, more and more people could learn to read."

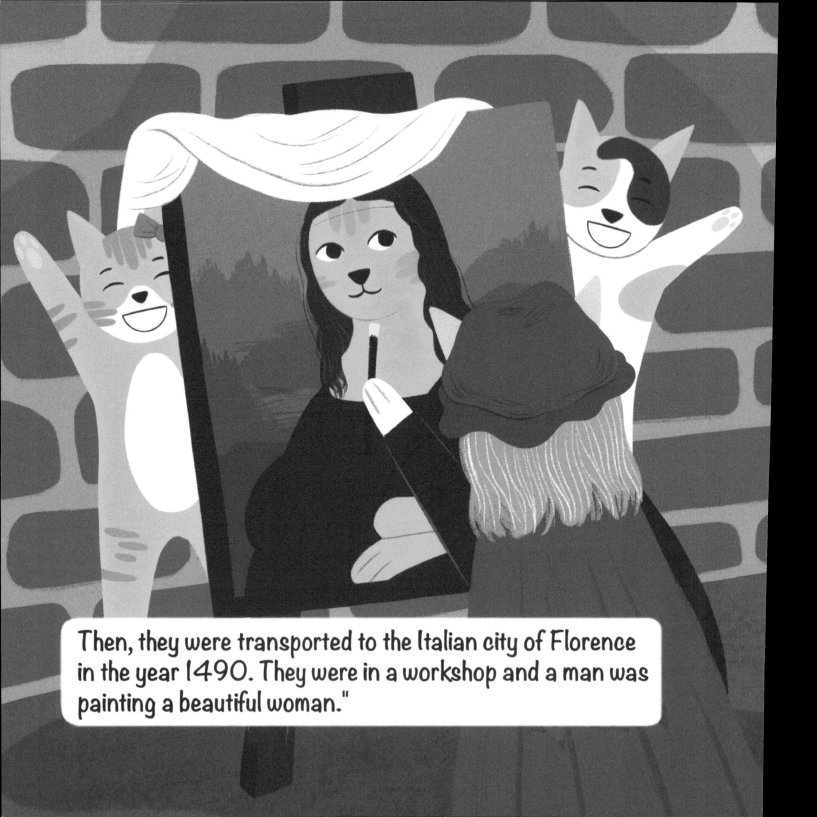

Then, they were transported to the Italian city of Florence in the year 1490. They were in a workshop and a man was painting a beautiful woman."

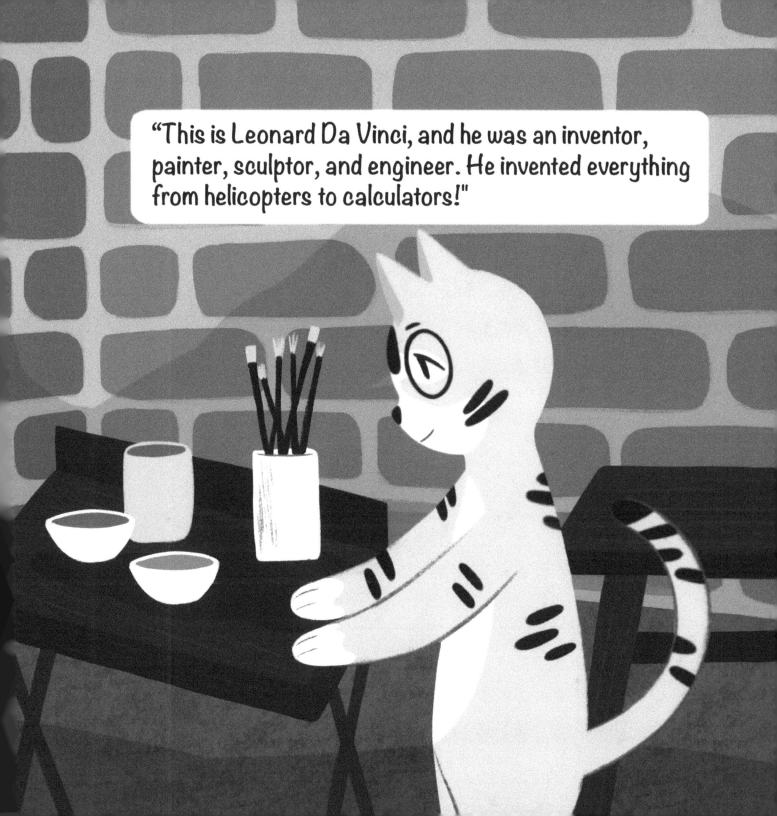

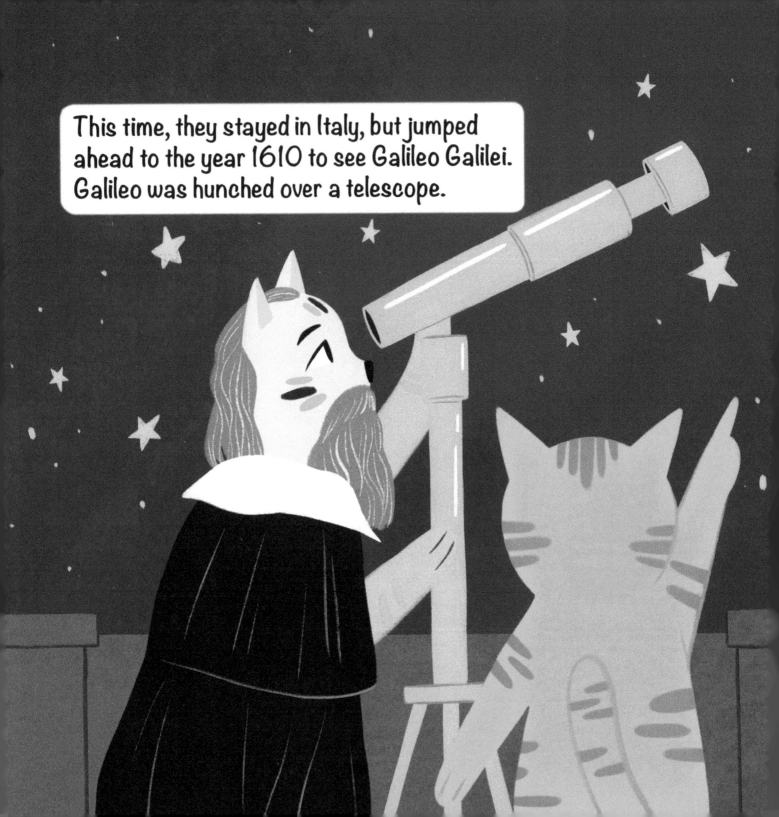

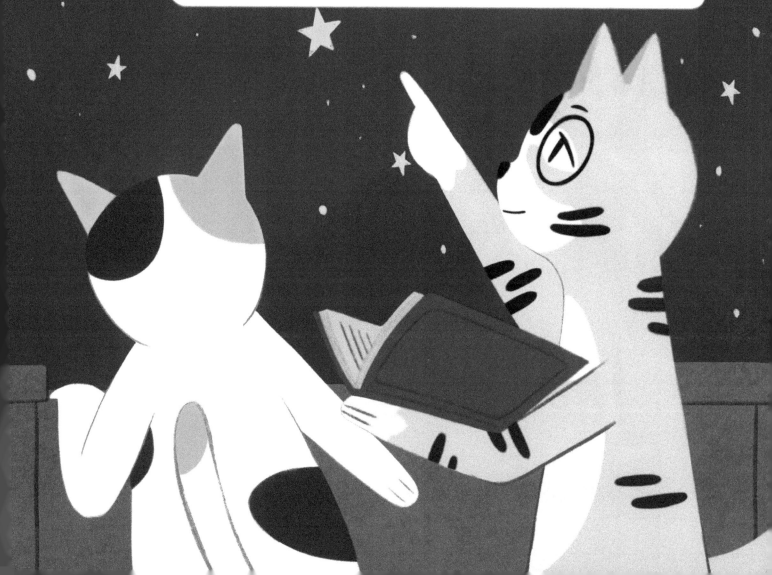

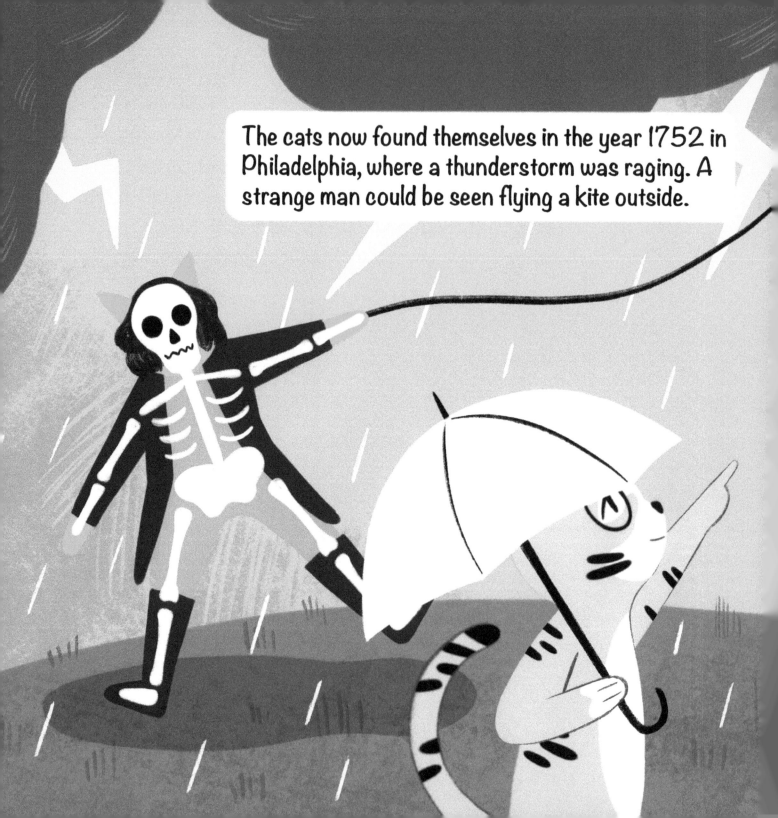

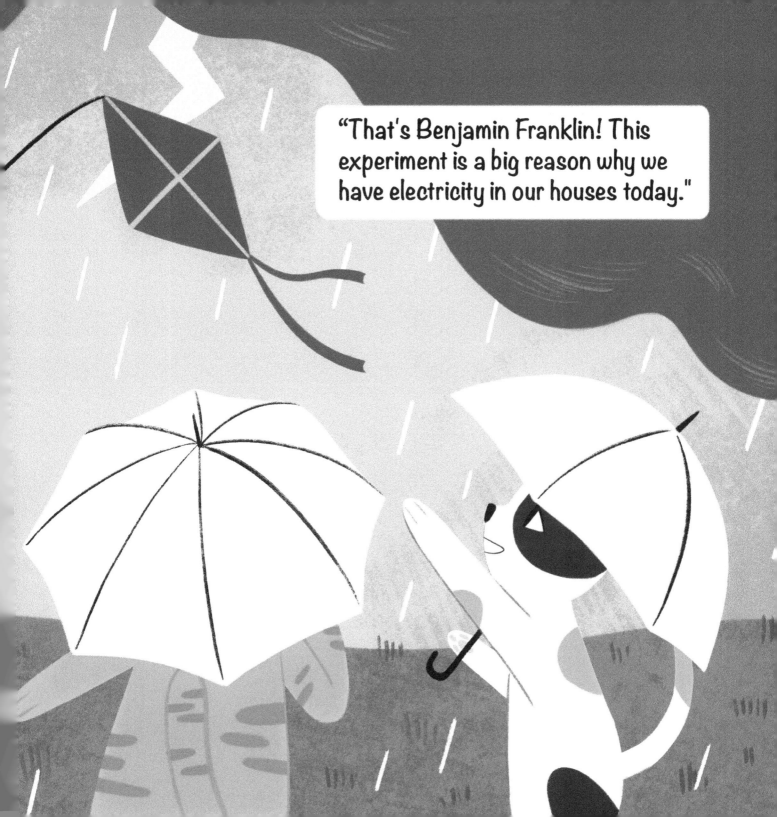

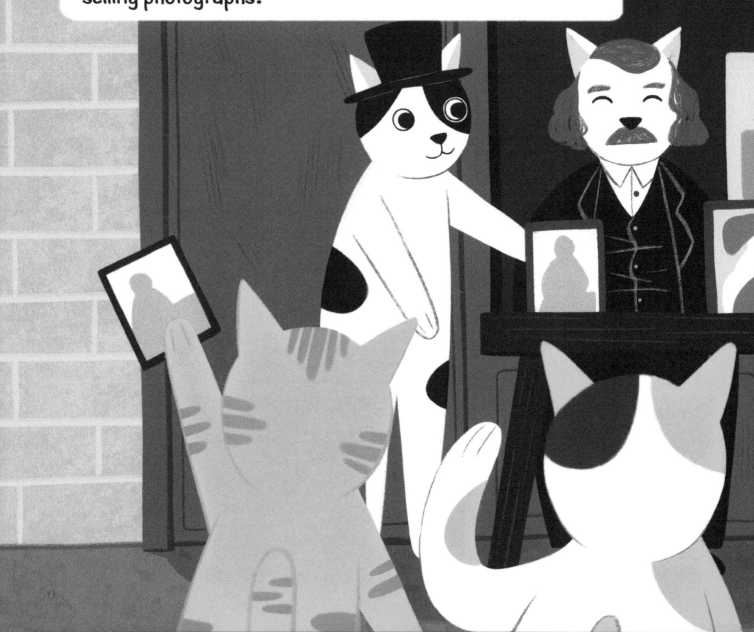

Now they zipped over to France in 1839. They were in a marketplace, and one shop was extremely crowded. It was selling photographs!

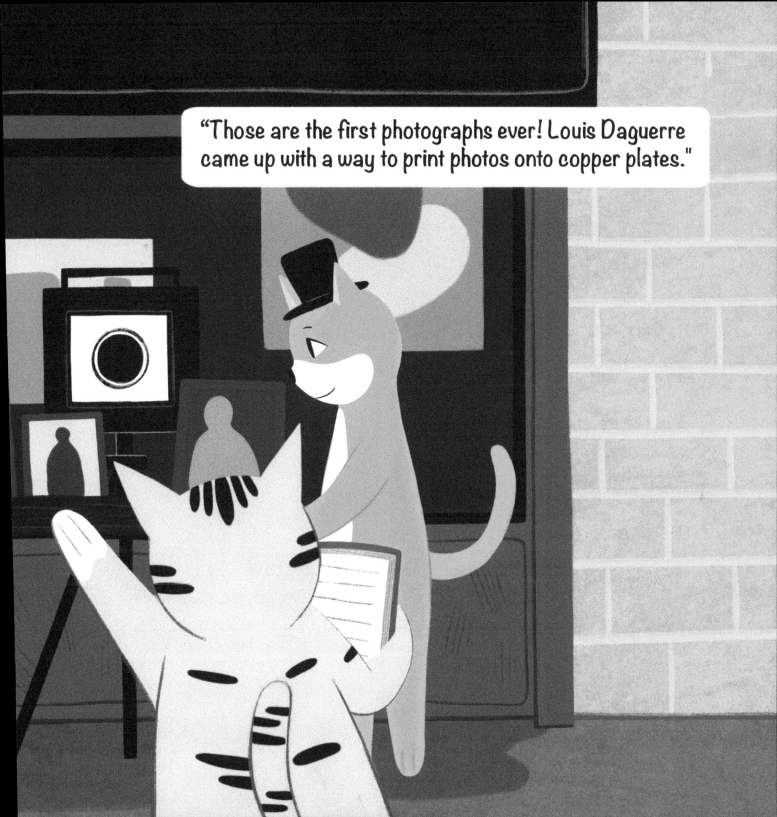

The cats headed to Boston in 1877 to see their next inventor. Alexander Graham Bell was publicly demonstrating his telephone.

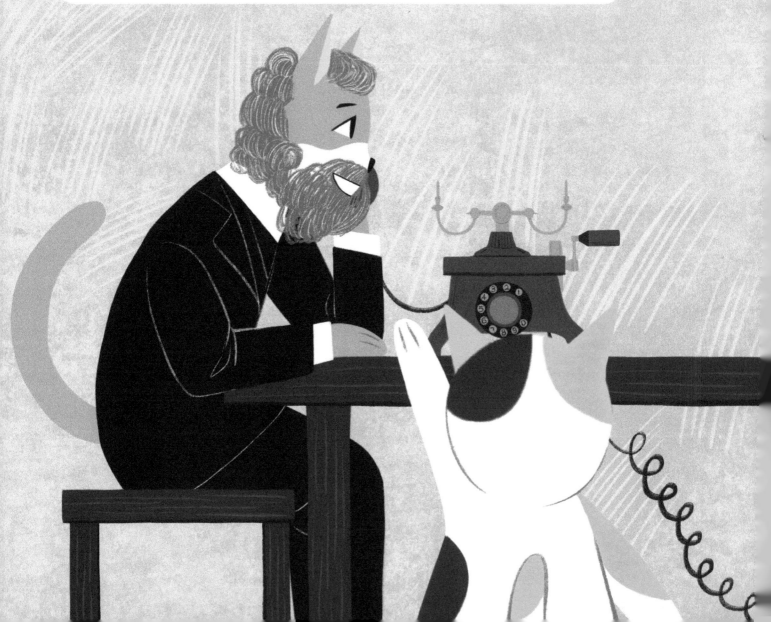

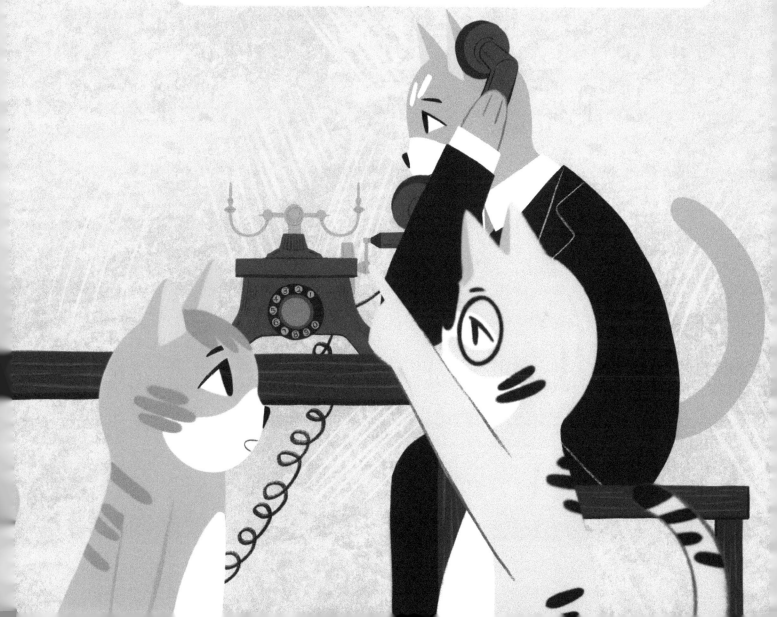

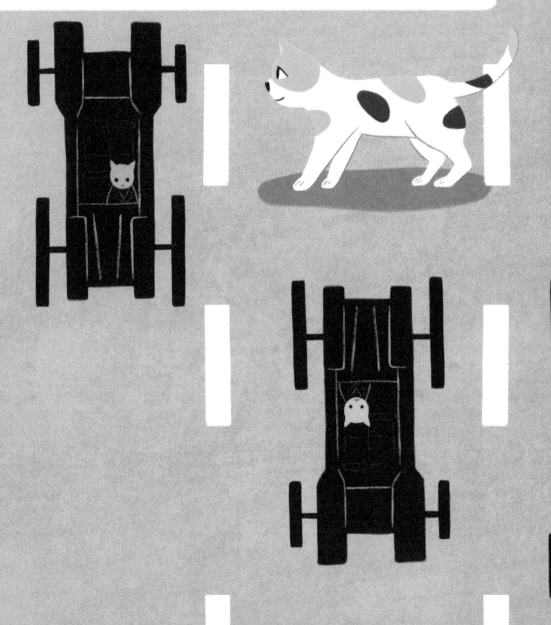

Next, these cats headed to Detroit in the year 1920. They could see some strange vehicles crowding the streets.

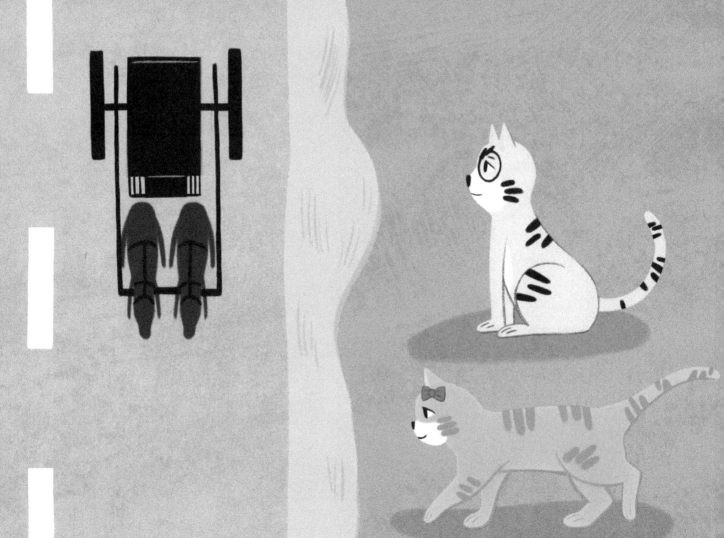

"Though these look quite different from the cars we have today, Henry Ford's car revolution started with these roofless cars with only one seat. If not for him, we would still be travelling around in horsecarts!"

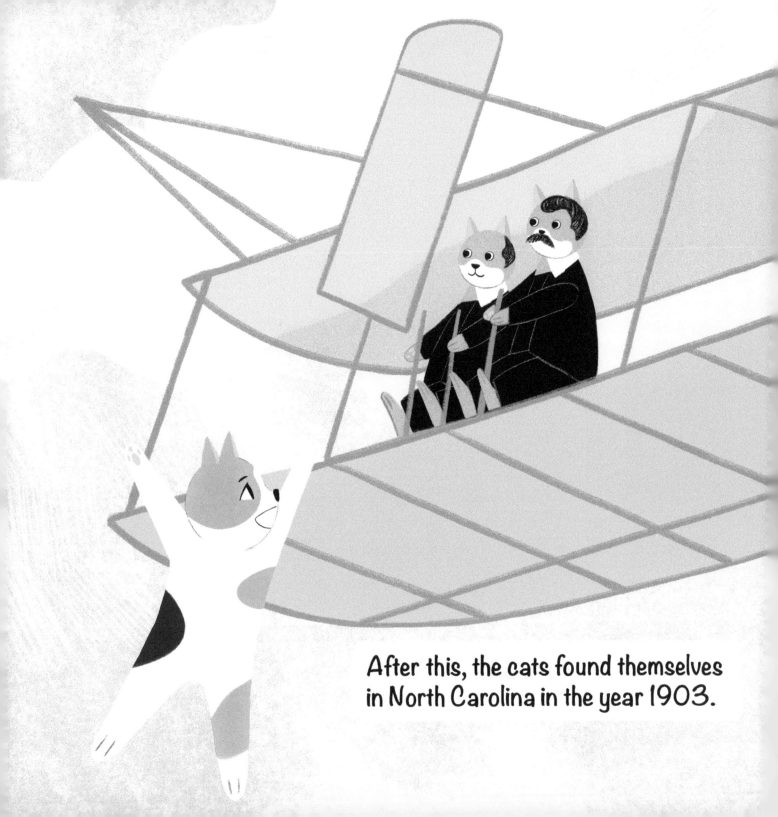

After this, the cats found themselves in North Carolina in the year 1903.

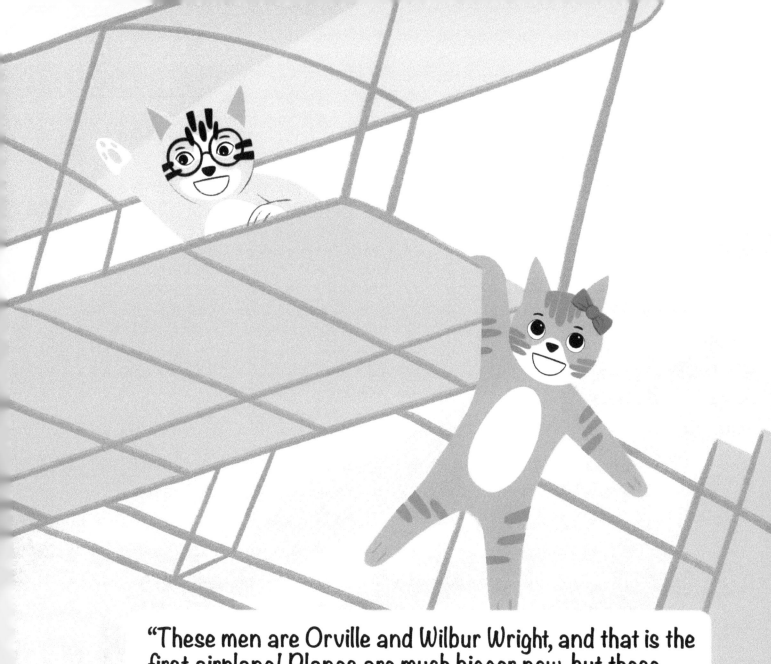

"These men are Orville and Wilbur Wright, and that is the first airplane! Planes are much bigger now, but these brothers made it possible for humans to fly in the sky."

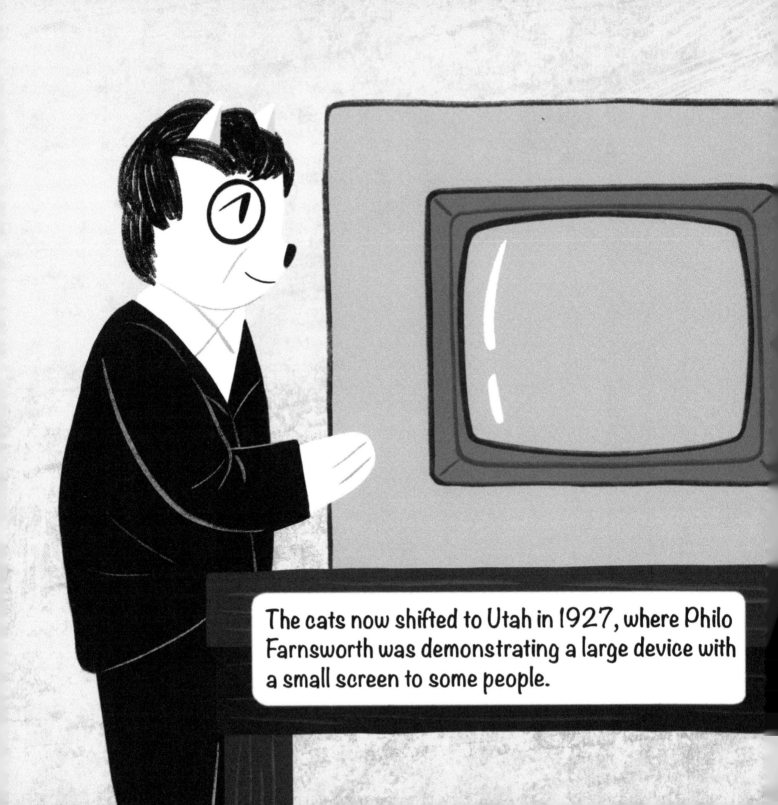

The cats now shifted to Utah in 1927, where Philo Farnsworth was demonstrating a large device with a small screen to some people.

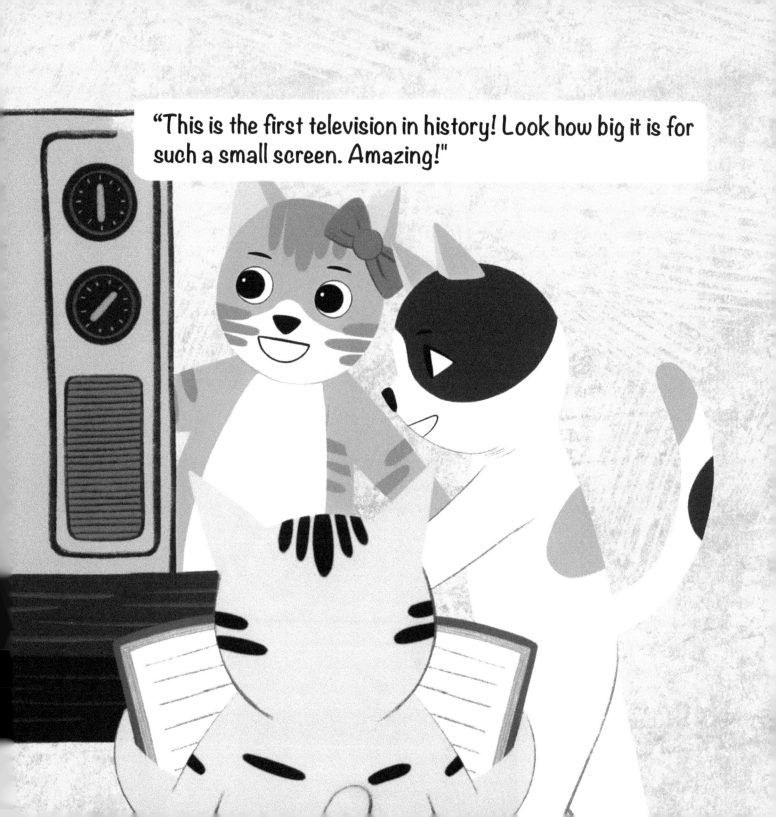

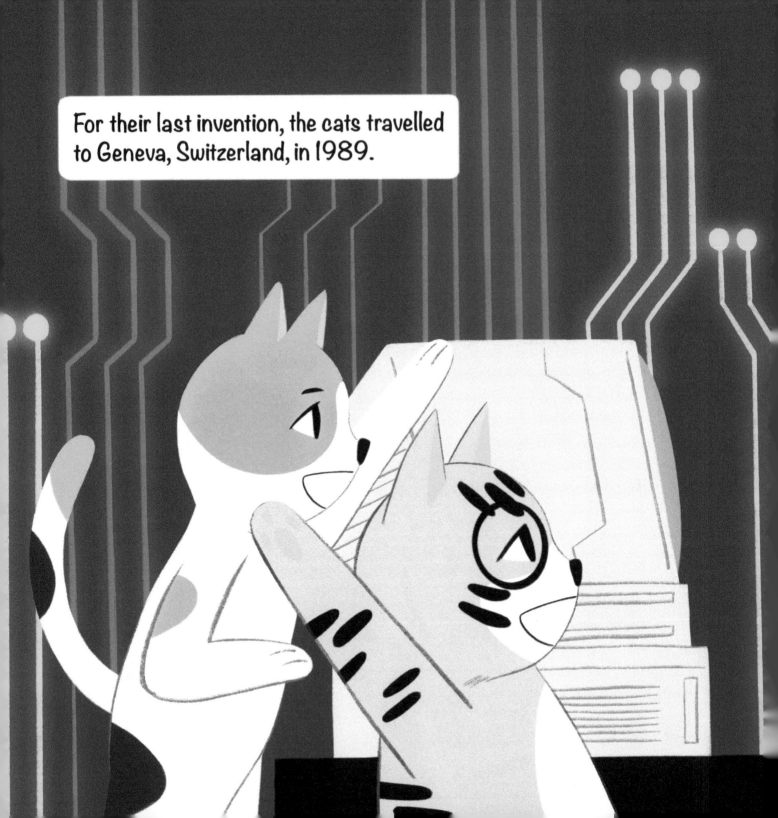

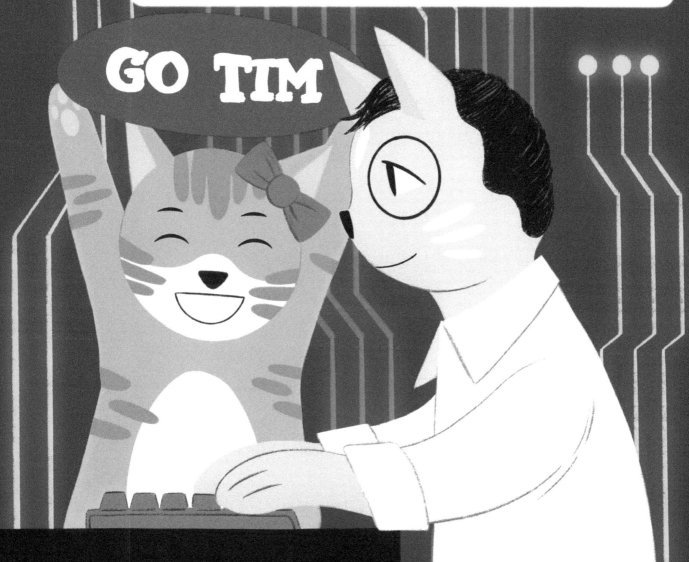

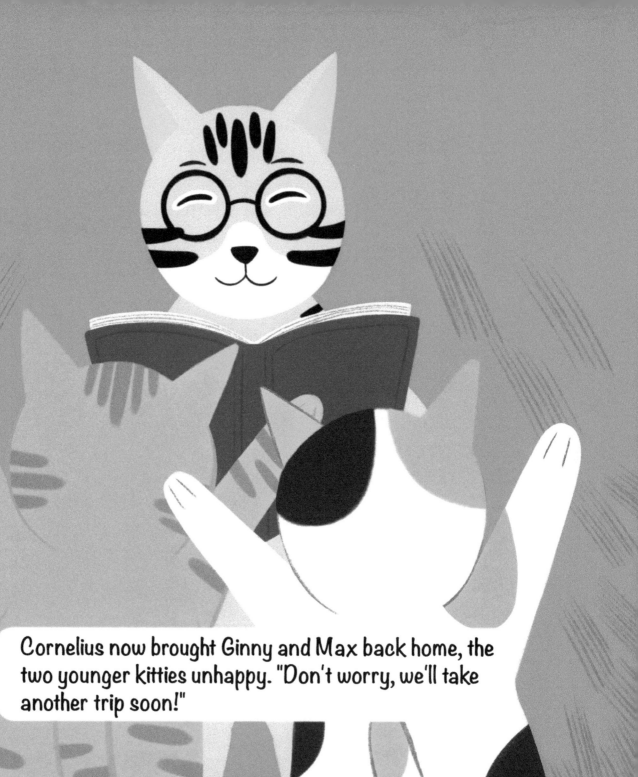

Cornelius now brought Ginny and Max back home, the two younger kitties unhappy. "Don't worry, we'll take another trip soon!"

Ginny and Max went back to playing with their toy cars. They wondered what they would learn next time!

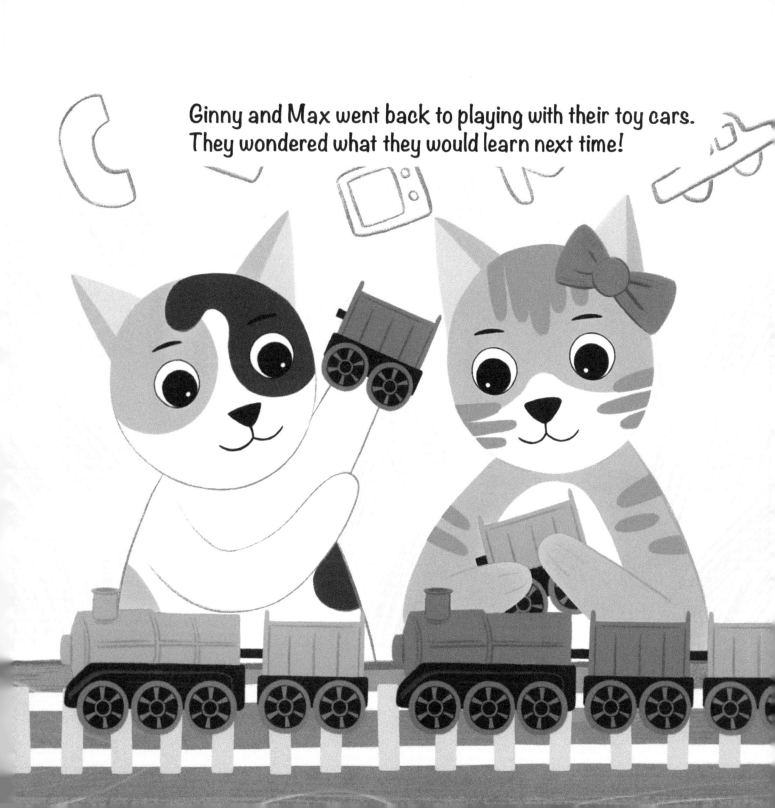

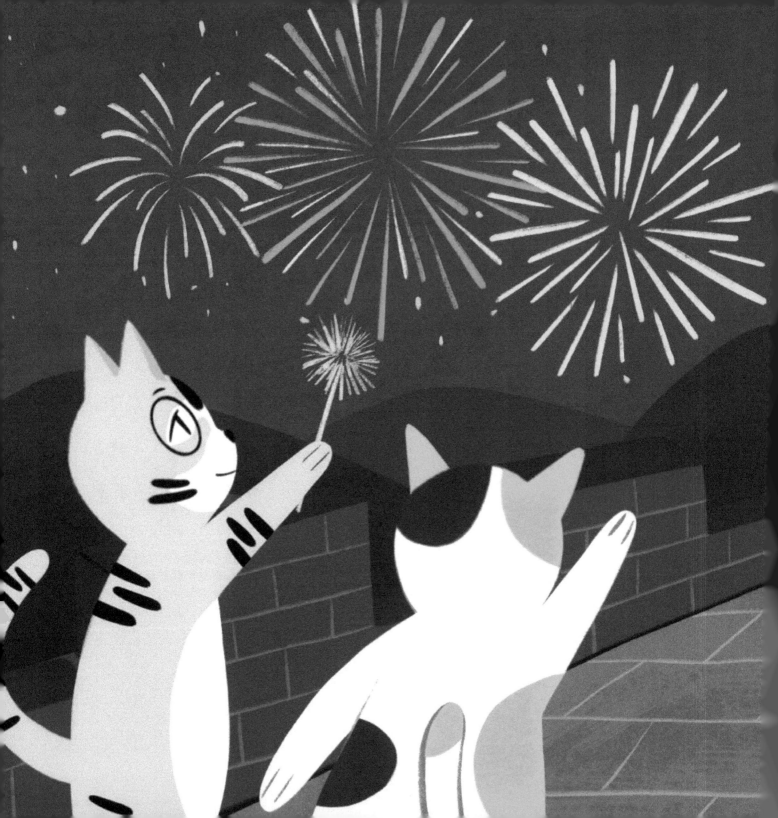

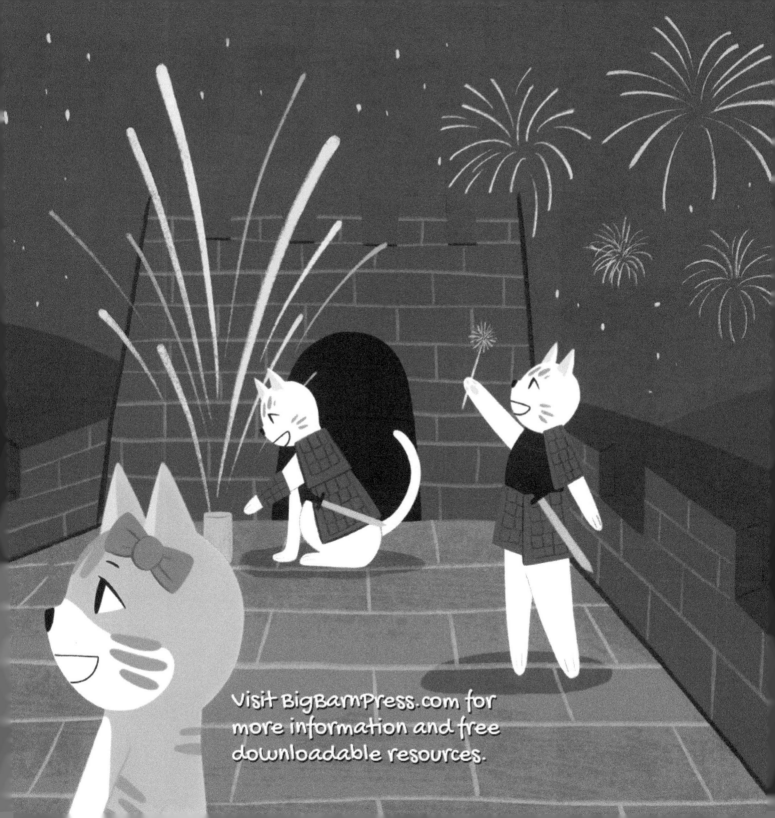

Visit BigBamPress.com for more information and free downloadable resources.

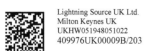

Lightning Source UK Ltd.
Milton Keynes UK
UKHW051948051022
409976UK00009B/203